Coconut Oil

Using Coconut Oil For Weight Loss, Increased Energy, Vibrant Beauty and Achieving Amazing Health

By Anne Wilson

2nd Edition

Table of Contents

Introduction

I want to thank you and congratulate you for purchasing the book, *"Coconut Oil: Using Coconut Oil For Weight Loss, Increased Energy, Vibrant Beauty and Achieving Amazing Health"*.

This book contains proven steps and strategies on how to use coconut oil in a number of ways so that you can reach your ideal weight goal, have more energy to do more things, look and feel more beautiful, and become healthier in general. .

Coconut oil has come a long way from being simply used as a cooking oil in the kitchen. It has now been found to have plenty of uses outside the realm of food and cooking, such as enhancing one's beauty, treating its health issues, and improving one's overall health. This boils down to the fact that coconut oil helps your body absorb the nutrients it needs more efficiently. Getting all the vitamins, minerals, and other nutrients that your body requires for optimal functioning results in effective health and weight management, increased desirability, and more energy, all of which coconut oil is able to deliver.

Thanks again for purchasing this book, I hope you enjoy it!

CHAPTER 1

Discovering an All-In-One Superfood

Coconut oil has been around, and has been in pantries all over the world, as both food and medicine. Research that has spanned throughout the past 50 years has proven that coconut oil contains special properties that allow it to be used in several important medical and nutritional applications.

Coconut palm has been a subject of research and documentation for about 4,000 years, and it is among the top fruits when it comes to providing benefits to consumers. It is also viewed as one of the more sustainable resource available to mankind because harvested materials that come from it impact almost every aspect of life, with the fruit being the most valuable since it's the source of coconut flesh, milk, water, and oil.

Coconut oil has been used in many cultures in tropical regions, which include Africa, the Indian subcontinent, Polynesia, majority of Asia, and Central and South America. Coconut oil has been an essential and documented part of Ayurvedic medicine. It's believed to be able to cure almost every area that relates to the body, mind, and spirit. The early European explorers marveled at how communities across the Pacific have made coconut oil part of almost every aspect of their daily lives. During World War II, coconut water has been used as a saline drop; and right after the war, England sold solid coconut oil as coconut butter or margarine.

In 1954, scientists discovered that unrefined virgin coconut oil is in fact healthier and more nutritious than most of the other oils being used as part of a household's diet. This made the coconut oil rise above the traditional notion that any oil that is rich in saturated fat is bad for one's health. However, research revealed that certain saturated fats are great for the body and are likely to promote good health when introduced to one's diet the right way.

While coconut oil had an awful reputation for being a source of saturated fat, it is also the source of the saturated fats that your body needs in order to achieve good health. Coconut oil contains medium-chain fatty acids, which is also found in abundance in human breast milk. Since these fatty acids are easily absorbed into the body, coconut oil improves the absorption of other nutrients one may derive from coconut and also improve the way the body receives energy.

Extracting Nature's Elixir

Coconut oil is typically extracted from the meat or kernel of a mature coconut. Virgin coconut oil is extracted from fresh coconuts, instead of copra (which is the source of most commercial coconut oil). Coconut oils derived from copra often need to be bleached, deodorized, and refined to be good enough for consumption.

If you have been using organic virgin coconut oil, you'll be glad to know that it's among the healthiest oils available. Virgin coconut oil comes from the fruit and is extracted and packaged without having to be deodorized and refined. Without the refinements, you can enjoy the many nutritional and antibacterial benefits that you can get out of this oil.

Debunking Myths about Coconut Oil

Various cultures, races, and religions revere the coconut. Wherever a coconut palm grows, people learn the importance of this crop as a very effective medicine. However, most people do rely on hearsay about food sources and the value that they offer. In order to truly understand how you can benefit from coconut oil, it will be best to debunk the myths surrounding this food product once and for all.

Myth: Coconut oil increases the risk of cardiovascular disease.

Fact: Coconut oil is predominantly made up of saturated fat, but there is no study that proves that coconut oil contributes to the rise of bad cholesterol in one's body. Coconut oil, however, raises the amount of good cholesterol, which lowers the amount of bad cholesterol and clears up arterial blockages.

Myth: Saturated fat in coconut oil leads to obesity.

Fact: What coconut oil does to the body is actually the opposite – the medium-chain fatty acids found in coconut oil's saturated fat content actually improve one's metabolism. That means that the body consumers and generates more energy, and that means fat stores are more likely be used. Coconut oil is also prescribed to people who want to lose weight. Having a system when it comes to taking in coconut oil will help you lose weight faster.

Myth: Coconut oil irritates the skin.

Fact: The truth is actually the exact opposite – coconut oil is proven to be one of the most soothing oils for the skin. It is also very effective when it comes to relieving irritation caused by allergies, sunburn, insect bites, and bruises. Coconut oil's antimicrobial properties can also help heal wounds faster.

Myth: The sweetness in coconut oil makes it bad for diabetics.

Fact: Coconut oil tastes like any other oil – it is definitely not sweet as it's made of pure fat. It does not contain any glucose. More importantly, coconut oil is known to promote the secretion of insulin to the pancreas, which is essential when it comes to controlling diabetes. In fact, regular use of coconut oil can greatly decrease the risk of acquiring diabetes later on in life.

Myth: Since coconut oil comes from coconut, which contains moisture, it can go rancid over a short amount of time.

Fact: This oil is so stable that despite holding some moisture, it still has a longer shelf life compared to other oils. Coconut oil does not go rancid for years, making it an ideal product to stock in the pantry.

Myth: Coconut oil tastes bad.

Fact: Everything is a matter of taste, but even the staunchest of critics is not likely to say that it has a foul taste. Since coconut oil tastes much like any other oil that you have in your pantry, the only thing that you need to do is to try it out for yourself.

Time to Discover the Magic

Now that you know how coconut oil can improve your life, it's time for you to discover how you can effectively use this superfood. The next chapters will show you how you can incorporate coconut oil in your daily life.

CHAPTER 2

Losing Excess Weight With Coconut Oil

Coconut oil used to get such a bad rap, mainly due to the findings of researchers who focused on how the hydrogenated variety affects your health. During the 1960s, most food manufacturers wanted consumers to buy margarine and commercial oils, which prompted them to discredit the food products that people have long been using in their households to prepare food. To do that, food producers maintained that any food rich in saturated fat, such as coconut oil, promotes obesity and cardiovascular diseases.

Coconut oil is indeed rich in saturated fat – saturated fat comprises 90% of the calories that is found in coconut oil. However, fast forward to the 2000s, studies began to show that there is no link between saturated fat and heart disease. As for the products marketed as healthier alternatives, well, they have actually been associated with increased risks of cancer, diabetes, and obesity. It is a good thing though that recent studies have proven that contrary to popular belief, coconut oil helps people lose weight and controls their appetite.

If you are using unrefined and organic coconut oil, then you are in for a number of health benefits.

How Coconut Oil Can Help You Lose Weight

The belief that coconut oil is bad for one's health was quickly reversed once health experts took it upon themselves to examine the health benefits of using coconut oil, particularly with regards to weight loss. They were able to identify a number of mechanisms by which coconut oil can help you succeed in your weight loss efforts.

What makes coconut oil different from most of the cooking oils used in households is that it has a unique composition of fatty acids. Not only does this make it ideal for high-heat cooking due to its resistance to oxidation on higher temperatures, the medium-chain triglycerides found in this oil also make a huge effect in the body's ability to produce energy without having to ingest more calories than necessary.

Coconut oil gives your metabolism a boost. Coconut oil contains abundant amounts of triglycerides called medium chain fatty acids (MFAs), which have the ability to improve a slow-moving metabolism. It has been identified in a certain study made on coconut oil that MFAs can raise the rate at which your metabolism runs by as much as almost fifty percent and for as long as twenty-four hours. Taking coconut oil on a daily basis can help you reverse the damage brought on by stress or dieting on your metabolism.

One of the essential properties of coconut oil is its being "thermogenic", which means that it tends to burn fat faster and improves energy expenditure. You will be expending more calories when you have coconut oil in your diet (compared to other fats). One to two teaspoons of coconut oil can increase your energy expenditure by about 120 calories in a single day.

Coconut oil controls your blood sugar levels. Even without the support of digestive enzymes, coconut oil can be easily absorbed in your body. This puts less stress on your pancreas and enables it to make insulin in a more efficient manner. Moreover, the fact that coconut oil is a type of saturated fat helps it bind more easily with insulin throughout the digestive process. Because your body is able to get the sufficient amount of insulin it needs, your cells are able to get the blood sugar (glucose) they require. This helps you control your appetite as well as curb your cravings, resulting in weight loss.

Coconut oil aids in stabilizing hormone levels. A number of your body's regular activities, such as thyroid function, digestion, and especially metabolism, are affected when your body does not get the fatty acids it requires to manufacture the hormones needed for these processes to take place. Coconut oil is able to convert your blood cholesterol into healthy hormones (a sterone called pregnenolone) that help improve your digestion as well as burn off any fat stores you may have around your thigh, buttock, and waist areas.

Coconut oil helps in curbing cravings and decreasing hunger. The medium-chain triglycerides, or MCTs, in coconut oil goes right into your liver during digestion, which promotes extended energy boost. At the same time, processed MCTs also promote ketone bodies that help reduce cravings and make you feel less hungry. Without needing to satisfy cravings and by staying energized throughout the day, you will find it easier to lose weight. While the notion that weight loss is all about burning more calories than you take in, it still holds a great amount of truth.

Although it's true that people need a calorie deficit in order to shed pounds, it does not mean that you have to consciously count calories or be too consciously aware about not eating. Since you have reduced appetite and that will lead to you unconsciously taking in fewer calories, you will immediately notice that coconut oil is taking effect. How does this happen? Medium-chain fatty acids make you feel full. This feeling fullness may be related to the way medium-chain fatty acids are metabolized by the body, which leads to the liver's production of ketone bodies. Ketone bodies are known to have a powerful effect when it comes to reducing appetite.

Here's a tip – if you want to eradicate the habit of snacking heavily in between meals and feel full faster when you eat, make it a point to have 2 to 3 servings of coconut oil every day.

Coconut oil aids in weight loss better than olive oil. If you are planning to lose weight, you should refrain from using olive oil – contrary to popular belief, this so-called "healthy oil" contains high amounts of monounsaturated fat, which is a fatty acid commonly found in body fat. In comparison to oils that contain monounsaturated fat, coconut oil is the better choice in hastening weight loss.

Coconut oil helps your body burn fat. If you want to reduce your calorie intake and lose weight fast without doing anything risky to your health, then you may have found the right diet partner. Because coconut oil improves your body's ability to break down food and absorb nutrients, you will be able to lessen the amount of food that you eat without feeling lethargic.

Tips on including coconut oil in your weight loss diet:

1. Use coconut oil as a healthy replacement for regular oils or fats. You can safely use it in its solid form (straight out of the jar), but if you prefer to have it in its liquefied state, simply let the coconut oil container stand in hot water prior to using it.

2. Taking coconut oil about thirty minutes before you take your meal can help you feel fuller and more satisfied afterwards, which definitely helps you to lose weight.

3. Remember that the daily recommended amount of coconut oil (if you prefer taking it by the spoon) for adults is one to three tablespoons.

How to Use Coconut Oil to Lose Weight

You can use coconut oil in a number of ways, especially in your kitchen, for you to be able to drop down to your ideal weight (or at least maintain your current weight). Begin by following these food preparation tips:

1. Incorporate coconut oil in your slimming smoothies.

This recipe for a delicious weight-friendly smoothie lets you enjoy one without the clumps of coconut oil.

Yummy Raspberry Smoothie

Ingredients:

Melted coconut oil (1 to 2 tablespoons);
Rolled oats (3 to 4 tablespoons);
Milk (3/4 cup);
Frozen raspberries (1 cup);
Vanilla extract/powder (1/2 teaspoon);
Heavy cream (1/4 cup); ground nutmeg (a dash);
Honey date (1 piece).

Directions: In a small bowl, mix the rolled oats, milk, vanilla extract/ powder, heavy cream, ground nutmeg, and honey date together. Stir well before leaving it to soak for about one hour to eight hours. Blend the soaked mixture in a food processor along with the frozen raspberries. Once the mixture turns smooth, add the coconut oil in small amounts to ensure that no clumps are formed. Serve in a tall glass.

2. *Make your sweet treats weight-friendly with coconut oil.*

If you are trying to lose weight but you're having a hard time staying away from desserts, then coconut oil can be an ingredient that will save you from the guilt. Here is a sneaky way for you to indulge in a sweet treat without wreaking havoc on your weight loss plan.

Decadent Coco Butter Cups

Ingredients:

Coconut oil (3 tablespoons);
Vanilla extract (1 tablespoon);
Shredded coconut (1 cup);
Gluten-free, dairy-free, and soy-free dark chocolate (1 pound);
Stevia extract (10 drops).

Directions: Place the coconut oil (2 tbsp), shredded coconut, vanilla extract, and stevia extract in a blender and process until well blended and the mixture turns out thick and smooth (with the consistency of almond butter). Let the coconut mixture stand while melting the chocolate in a bowl placed inside a small pot filled with boiling water. Add the rest of the coconut oil (1 tbsp); once melted, pour half of the melted chocolate and coconut oil mixture into silicon muffin cups (ensure that the sides of the muffin cups are coated by rotating them). Transfer the filled muffin cups in the freezer to allow them to set. Once hardened, remove from the freezer and fill each cup with one tablespoon of the prepared coconut mixture (to flatten, gently press down using the back of a spoon). Top the coconut mixture with the remaining chocolate and coconut oil mixture, and then return to the freezer to set. Once completely hardened, take out of the muffin cups and serve immediately (or keep in an airtight jar).

3. Use coconut oil as a healthy stand-in for unhealthy fats when baking.

Coconut oil is ideal for cooking, especially since it can withstand high temperatures. In fact, it is commonly used in baking. Coconut oil is a good substitute for margarine, butter, and vegetable oils in most baking recipes, such as the following:

Coconut Oil Chicken Roast

Ingredients:

Melted coconut oil (1/4 cup);
water (2 tablespoons);
quartered small yellow onion (1 piece);
chicken stock (1/2 cup);
halved garlic cloves (4 pieces);
corn starch (1 ½ tablespoons);
melted grass-fed butter (1/4 cup);
sea salt (a pinch + a handful);
freshly ground pepper (a dash + a handful);
garlic powder (1/2 teaspoon);
celery (1 stalk); and chicken (1 whole).

Directions: Set the oven at 425 degrees to preheat. After removing the giblets and washing in warm tap water, dry the chicken thoroughly. Use a handful each of pepper and salt to season the cavity before stuffing with the garlic, celery, and onion. Use a brush to coat all sides of the chicken with the coconut oil and melted grass-fed butter, then season all over with the garlic powder and the remaining pepper and salt. Set the seasoned chicken in a large roasting pan and place in the oven to roast for about eleven minutes. Lower the heat (down to 350 degrees) before basting the chicken, and then allow to roast for one hour, by which time its juices should run clear when pierced between the thigh and leg. Use the pan juices to baste the chicken every ten to fifteen minutes (except the last ten minutes); transfer the remaining pan juices to a saucepan heated over medium-low heat and add in the chicken stock. Meanwhile, combine the corn starch with the water, then pour into the saucepan. Whisk well while bringing to a gentle boil. Once the gravy has thickened, serve alongside your roasted chicken.

4. Enhance the flavor of your fried foods with coconut oil.

If you have had trouble using other healthy oils in frying because of their limited capacity to withstand high temperatures, coconut oil will be ideal to use. It's a less decadent alternative to the refined cooking oils that you might be using in your kitchen. This satisfying shrimp recipe lets you try using coconut oil in your fried dishes:

Delicious Coconut Shrimp

Ingredients:

Coconut oil (1 to 2 cups);
Almond flour (1 cup);
Sea salt (1 tablespoon + 1 teaspoon);
Eggs (2 pieces);
Garlic powder (1 teaspoon);
Pepper (1 teaspoon);
Thinly shredded unsweetened coconut (1 cup);
Shrimp (1 pound);
Water (1 teaspoon);
Honey (2 tablespoons).

Directions: In a skillet heated on medium-high, pour the coconut oil. Meanwhile, peel and de-vein the shrimp with their tails on. In a large bowl, combine the eggs, water, salt (1 tsp), pepper, and garlic powder by beating well. In a separate bowl, stir the almond flour and shredded coconut together. Douse each shrimp into the egg mixture before coating with the flour mixture, and then fry in the heated oil for about three minutes on each side. Sprinkle with the remaining salt (1 tablespoon) before serving.

CHAPTER 3

Gaining More Energy With Coconut Oil

Most people nowadays live with the truth that stress and fatigue is already part of life, and that coffee isn't enough anymore. For people who want the right pick-me-up without having to rely on strong energy drinks that come with increased caloric intake, coconut oil is going to be a great natural alternative.

The fact that the fatty acids found in coconut oil are immediately used as fuel for the body's energy, rather than being put into storage like other types of fats, provide a number of benefits. First among them is the energy boost that you get – it's not similar to the kick that caffeine gives you; rather, it is more subtle but lasts longer. Moreover, the boosting effect that it provides is cumulative, meaning that you get more energized through continued use.

How Coconut Oil Can Help Increase Your Energy

Coconut oil is the right choice when it comes to finding the type of fat that lets you naturally increase your energy, which also makes it a great alternative to snacking on food items that are rich in calories when you need to keep yourself awake and energized for an extended amount of time. A number of reasons enable coconut oil to give you the energy boost you need:

Your body is able to digest coconut oil easily. Other kinds of oils and fats have to be processed by your body with the help of your pancreas' digestive enzymes as well as your gallbladder's bile, whereas coconut oil does not require these substances in order to be digested. Instead of placing added stress on your digestive system, the medium chain fatty acids of coconut oil are directly transported to and converted into useable energy in your liver. Moreover, the fact that coconut oil is easily digested by your body helps the latter conserve the energy it will have used in digesting other types of oils and fats.

Your body does not store coconut oil as body fat. Other types of oils and fats contain low chain fatty acids that are not easily digested by your body. They bind to protein and cholesterol once inside your body, after which they are circulated while releasing small fat particles along the way. These fat particles are then added to your fat stores. Meanwhile, the medium chain fatty acids in coconut oil are not stored along with your body fat; instead, they are easily converted into energy and help increase your metabolism rate, which further gives you an energy boost.

Your body is able to absorb nutrients more easily through coconut oil. Coconut oil will help you get the most nutrients out of your meals, especially the mineral magnesium (found in brown rice, kelp, spinach, seeds, nuts, and beans) and the B vitamins (found in whole grains, vegetables, and fresh fruits), which your body requires in order to produce energy.

Who Uses Coconut Oil for Energy

If you are wondering whether you can incorporate coconut oil in your diet, think about this – if you regularly consume energy drinks, then you definitely have the time and resources to take advantage of this natural alternative. It shouldn't cost much more than those beverages and it isn't too complicated to take either. Coconut oil will prove to be beneficial to the following:

1. People who do sports

If you need to enhance your endurance, stamina, and performance, it would be best to incorporate coconut oil in your diet.

2. People who live busy and unhealthy lives

Today, it is possible for people to get caught in a highly stressful environment which may trap them into living an extremely unhealthy lifestyle, making them prone to physical and mental stress. If you feel fatigued too often, then it may be best to give yourself some push with coconut oil.

3. Elderly people with limiting diet

People who are in the later years of their lives may have to limit their food intake. Coconut oil can help them get enough energy even with dietary restrictions in place.

Tips on including coconut oil in your energy-boosting diet:

1. Coconut oil may be good for your health, but it does contain calories (9 per gram). You still have to consider the amount of calories your body takes in whenever you consume coconut oil for its energy-boosting benefits. Otherwise, you could end up gaining weight (an undesirable result that can also zap your energy).

2. Don't simply add coconut oil to all your dishes. Instead, use it as a substitute for your cooking oils or fats. Using coconut oil for frying will also help you cook better since it can withstand higher temperatures.

How to Use Coconut Oil to Increase Your Energy

You may already be convinced of coconut oil's ability to give you added energy, but if you are having second thoughts about taking it due to its texture or flavor, there are ways for you to including it in your diet without letting its distinct taste and texture overpower your taste buds:

1. Add coconut oil to your morning coffee.

Drinking your daily cup of hot coffee in the morning is a perfect way of consuming coconut oil to increase your energy levels. Dealing with its oily consistency can put you off though; fortunately, this recipe will allow coconut oil to lend well into your coffee and let you come up with rich and creamy brew.

Perk-Me-Up Coffee

Ingredients: Coconut oil (1 to 2 tablespoons); organic coffee/herbal coffee/chai tea (1 cup); vanilla (1/4 teaspoon); unsalted grass-fed butter (1 teaspoon); and stevia extract (2 drops).

Directions: Pour the organic coffee/herbal coffee/chai tea into a blender. Add the coconut oil, vanilla, butter, and stevia extract. Process on high for about twenty seconds or until the mixture turns out frothy. Drink and enjoy right away.

2. Enhance the taste of homemade energy bars with coconut oil.

For those who rely on added energy, making an energy bar that incorporates coconut oil is among the smartest (and tastiest) things to do. Bursting with healthy fats and energy-boosting benefits, this recipe for coconut energy bars will be a sure hit among kids and adults alike.

Coconut Bars

Ingredients:

Coconut oil (1/2 cup);
Chia seeds/thinly shredded coconut (1/2 cup);
Cocoa powder (1/2 cup);
Shredded coconut (1 1/5 cups);
Stevia extract (2 drops);
Cocoa butter (1/2 cup);
Vanilla extract (2 drops).

Directions: Heat a small saucepan on low. Add the cocoa butter and allow it to melt, before adding the coconut oil. Stir well and then add the honey, cocoa powder, and chia seeds/thinly shredded coconut. Add the vanilla and stevia extracts before pouring the mixture into a baking dish (9x13) lined with parchment paper. Place in the refrigerator for about one hour to set, before cutting into bars. Serve and enjoy.

3. Kick up the energy-boosting factor of protein shakes with coconut oil.

Take your protein shakes to the next energy-giving levels by following this simple recipe:

Choco Coconut Banana Protein Shake

Ingredients:

Melted coconut oil (1 to 3 tablespoons);
Cocoa (1 teaspoon);
Raw organic whole milk/coconut milk (1/2 cup);
Guar gum (1/4 teaspoon);

Xantham gum (1/4 teaspoon);
Frozen banana (1 piece);
Chocolate-flavored protein powder (2 to 3 scoops);
Ice cubes (5 pieces);
Water (3/4 cup).

Directions: In a blender, pour the whole milk/coconut milk and water. Add the guar gum, xantham gum, frozen banana, protein powder, and ice cubes. Process well while gradually adding the coconut oil. Once the texture becomes smooth, pour into a tall glass and drink immediately.

4. Incorporate coconut oil in hot drinks.

Besides adding it to your hot coffee, you can also use coconut oil to "power up" other hot drinks. Try this recipe for hot milk:

Choco Pecan Milk

Ingredients:

Virgin coconut oil (3 tablespoons);
Organic cocoa powder (2 tablespoons);
Pecans (1/4 cup);
Hot organic whole milk (1 ½ cups);
Raw honey (1 to 2 tablespoons).

Directions: Pour the hot milk in a food processor. Add the cocoa powder, pecans, and honey before blending well until the mixture is smooth. Gradually add the coconut oil into the food processor while letting it run. Serve in a large glass or mug.

5. Sneak in coconut oil in other ways:

Popcorn

Directions: Take a large pot (heavy-bottomed) and completely coat its surface with 2 tablespoons of coconut oil. Add ½ cup of popcorn, shaking the pot to make sure all the kernels are covered in coconut oil. Heat the pot on medium-high. Cover the pot, but allow the steam to escape by leaving the lid slightly open. Allow 5 minutes for the popcorn to completely pop.

Veggies

Directions: In a small bowl, combine coconut oil (1 tbsp), lemon juice (1 tbsp), thyme (1 tsp), salt (1 tsp), and pepper (1 tsp). Brush the resulting mixture on zucchini, butternut squash, sweet potatoes, beets, and other vegetables.

Sweet Potato Chips

Directions: Set the oven at 400 degrees to preheat. Meanwhile, cut the sweet potatoes into 1/8-inch-thick slices, and then place on a large baking sheet. Lightly brush the sweet potato slices with coconut oil before placing in the oven to bake for fifteen minutes or until they are lightly browned. Season with some salt and eat the sweet potato chips plain or with salsa.

Nut Butter

Directions: Place 2 cups of almonds, cashews, or another type of nuts in a food processor. Add coconut oil (2 tablespoons) and blend until the mixture turns out buttery-smooth. Add more flavor by drizzling a bit of maple syrup or honey, or adding a dash of cinnamon or ground coffee. You can use your nut butter as a delicious spread on your toast, bagel, or muffin for breakfast.

CHAPTER 4

Taking Beauty To The Next Level With Coconut Oil

There are few beauty products today that can provide solutions to almost every cosmetic concern, but coconut oil comes close to achieving this feat. Coconut oil can be used for almost everything – from improving your nails, to softening your hair. Its affordability is just a bonus, given how versatile it is.

How Coconut Oil Can Help You Achieve Vibrant Beauty

Coconut oil allows you to achieve the vibrant beauty you have always desired to have by making your skin and hair healthier.

Soft and nourished skin. Your skin can benefit from coconut oil's moisturizing benefits, making it naturally nourished and hydrated. Coconut oil has the ability to replenish the oils in your skin with the medium chain type of fatty acids it contains, which even have antibacterial, antifungal, and antiviral properties that help make your skin healthy. Bad bacteria, fungi, and toxins can build up on your skin, causing it to suffer from dehydration and other problems. What coconut oil does is that it helps cleanse your skin of these skin-damaging agents; it also neutralizes them, so your skin's outer layer is detoxified as well as protected.

Coconut oil may also be the only moisturizer that you would want to use from now on. Not only does it save you from having dehydrated skin (protecting it from fungi, bacteria, and toxins that you may encounter on a daily basis), it's also easy to apply. Since the body's temperature is typically above 97°F, your skin will easily absorb coconut oil. This means that there is no greasy feeling after use.

Coconut oil is typically solid at room temperature, which will allow you to store and use this beauty product like petroleum jelly. However, it will stay liquid in higher temperatures and will melt once applied to the skin. Since coconut oil is a non-comedogenic substance, it will not leave any residues that could end up blocking pores.

Lush and glowing hair. Coconut oil can often be seen included in the list of ingredients of a number of hair cleansers and conditioners, and for a good reason: Coconut oil has the ability to penetrate deep within your hair shaft, allowing it to work on your hair more efficiently to make it shiny and vibrant.

How to Use Coconut Oil to Achieve Vibrant Beauty

<u>SKIN</u>

1. Fresh face

Cleansing your face with coconut oil might be the best thing you can do keep it healthy, glowing, and young-looking. Not only is coconut oil naturally moisturizing, antibacterial, and antibacterial in nature, it has also been identified by research studies to be beneficial for atopic dermatitis (a number of women have disclosed using coconut oil as a facial moisturizer at night). You can use coconut oil as part of a two-step face cleansing method (this technique works on skin that is not allergic to coconut oil and prone to adult-acne). With your fingers, gently rub and massage coconut oil over the skin on your face as well as on the neck, making sure to work in circular motions. Afterwards, use your favorite facial cleanser to wash off any residue.

2. Makeup-free eyes

Use coconut oil to remove your eye makeup. Cleansing your eyes of eye shadow, eyeliner, and even waterproof mascara becomes much easier on you (and less traumatic on your eyes) with the aid of a bit of coconut oil. Do note though, that it's more than capable of removing makeup in other areas as well. It's an excellent grease cutter and works even better than most commercial skin-cleaning products. In fact, many of such products contain a coconut-based detergent agent called sodium lauryl sulfate, which is powerful enough to remove grease and motor oil, yet gentle and safe enough for baby's skin.

Simply dip a cotton ball in a small amount of coconut oil, and then use it to wipe your eyelids as well as the under-eyes lightly. Coconut oil can effectively break down the wax and ink components of your eye makeup while leaving your delicate eye area hydrated. Afterwards, simply wash your face as you normally would. If you are going to use coconut oil to remove makeup from the rest of your face, you can use a cotton ball dabbed in coconut oil. Leave the oil on your face for about 5 minutes and then wash it off with gentle soap and warm water. While most of the makeup will be gone, you should reapply coconut oil on your face for deeper and thorough cleaning.

3. Smooth hands

Soothe your dry hands with the help of coconut oil's amazing moisturizing property. Using the oil can be messy if you are at work, but you can always take advantage of its skin hydrating benefits in the comfort of your home, especially after doing your dishwashing and other skin moisture-robbing chores. Just head to your kitchen, scoop up some coconut oil (solid or melted), and rub on your parched hands. Compared to several commercial moisturizers, coconut oil can easily be absorbed by the skin, leaving your hands moisturized without the stickiness.

4. Smooth legs

Beautiful, hair-free legs are easy to achieve even without your expensive traditional shaving creams, which are harmful to your skin anyway due to the chemicals they contain. Use coconut oil to prep your legs (as well as underarms) before shaving them. Coconut oil leaves your legs protected from microbes, smelling pleasant, feeling hydrated, and looking smooth.

5. Smooth body

Smoother skin all over your body is just an arm's length away, thanks to coconut oil. Stop wasting your money on commercial body scrubs. You can make your own inexpensive, homemade, fragrant, and chemical-free body scrub with the help of some ingredients already available in your kitchen. In a small saucepan heated on low, put ½ cup of coconut oil and allow it to melt. Once melted, let the melted coconut oil sit for one minute to cool, and then pour over 1 cup of salt or brown sugar. Use a spoon to stir the mixture while gradually adding in about 5 drops of lavender essential oil or pure vanilla extract.

6. Relaxed body

Treat yourself to some rubdown with the help of coconut oil. Many massage oils available in the market actually use coconut oil for their base. You can skip going to the store and buying another bottle of expensive massage oil. Simply pour some coconut oil on your hands and allow your body to feel relaxed and moisturized after a good rubdown.

7. Hydrated body

Coconut oil works as a great body moisturizer as well. A study done on animals on the use of coconut oil has shown that applying virgin coconut oil directly on the skin can actually help wounds heal faster. Meanwhile, a study done on humans on the same subject has demonstrated coconut oil's ability to effectively increase skin hydration as well as decrease the amount of moisture lost in severely dry skin.

8. Sun-protected body

Protect the skin all over your body from the sun by slathering on your own homemade sunscreen lotion. Try this recipe for making your coconut oil-infused sun-protector (coconut oil naturally has a sun protection factor, or SPF, of 4):

Skin-Friendly Sunscreen

Ingredients:

Coconut oil (1/4 cup);
Zinc oxide (2 tablespoons);
Beeswax (1/4 cup);
Olive oil/almond oil (1/2 cup);
Vitamin E oil (1 teaspoon);
Shea butter (2 tablespoons);
Raspberry seed oil (1 teaspoon);
Carrot seed oil (1 teaspoon);
Vanilla extract (5 drops).

Directions: In a large glass jar, mix together the coconut oil, olive oil/ almond oil, vitamin E oil, raspberry seed oil, and carrot seed oil. Stir in the beeswax, shea butter, and vanilla extract and then set aside. Meanwhile, heat a large saucepan filled with about two inches of water on medium-high. Loosely cover the jar containing the sunscreen mixture and place in the water-filled pan. Allow the ingredients to gradually melt as the water gets heated, stirring occasionally so that the mixture is well-blended. Once done, stir in the zinc oxide and then transfer into a clean mason jar. Give the mixture several stirs to incorporate the zinc oxide, before covering the jar. Use your homemade sunscreen within 6 months.

Take note though, that since coconut oil only comes with SPF 4, it will not be able to completely protect you from all the harmful effects of the sun. However, applying coconut oil on your skin before stepping out of the house will protect you from solar radiation. Should you ever spend the day under the sun without any protection, you can reduce any skin damage by applying coconut oil as soon as you can. Remember that the sun's ultraviolet rays can damage the skin, triggering the formation of free radicals that may harm cellular DNA in the long run. The antioxidants found in coconut oil can diminish the stress caused by oxidation, preventing reactions that may stem from this. In addition, coconut oil has a soothing effect when applied to burnt skin, which enables you to get immediate relief from the pain caused by spending too much time under the sun.

9. Antibacterial shield for the skin

Coconut oil's antibacterial properties are useful when it comes to protecting the skin from pathogens that you encounter every day. At the same time, these properties also allow you to protect yourself from exacerbating existing skin problems, such as acne. With lauric acid as one of the antibacterial compounds that exist in coconut oil, you can be sure that you will be keeping secondary bacteria (those that tend to proliferate in pus) under control.

10. Reduced facial wrinkles

If you want to preserve your youthful look and make sure that your face is wrinkle-free, then you have found the right product. Collagen, the protein that is located within the inner layers of the skin, is responsible for keeping one's skin smooth and elastic. However, this protein can be destroyed by being exposed to UV rays, smoking, injuries, and pollution. In order to maintain the skin's elasticity and smoothness, collagen must be replaced as soon as possible.

Because coconut oil has the ability to penetrate deep into the skin, the triglycerides found in the oil is able to attract protein molecules and ensure that collagen is replenished in a timely manner.

HAIR

1. Deep-conditioned tresses

Deep-condition your hair with coconut oil – its MCFAs (medium chain fatty acids) are able to work deeper into and faster on your hair because of their small size. For this reason, coconut oil can provide deep hydration to your scalp, repair your split ends, and make your hair strands glow with long-lasting shine, especially when used as an overnight hair treatment.

<u>Coconut Oil Deep Conditioner</u>

Materials:

Coconut oil, virgin, organic (1 jar);
Small bowl;
Large bowl;
Small towel or shower cap;
Hair pick or comb.

Directions: After carefully shampooing your hair, allow it to air-dry as you start working on your homemade deep conditioner. Use a spoon to scoop out some coconut oil into the small bowl, and then place the bowl inside the larger one. Pour hot water into the larger bowl so that the outside of the smaller bowl is half-submerged. Let the coconut oil melt and then dip your fingers into it. With gentle stroking motions, massage the heated coconut oil into your hair strands. Allow the oil to penetrate into the hair by working the hair pick or comb into the strands. Once all hair strands are fully coated with the oil, use the small towel or shower cap to cover your hair. Let the oil soak for half an hour or more before shampooing. You can reapply some coconut oil onto your clean hair strands afterwards for added shine.

2. Detangled strands

Coconut oil works effectively as a hair detangler, especially if you have long hair or have curly, unmanageable strands. What is great about using coconut oil to tame your tresses is that it does not leave any unwanted residue that can weigh down your hair and make it difficult to style. Plus, coconut oil as a natural hair detangler does not expose your hair strands to any long-term damage. Try this easy recipe for your own hair detangler – it will make styling your long hair or brushing your curly strands a breeze:

Coconut Oil Hair Detangler

Materials:

A jar of virgin coconut oil (organic);
A hairbrush;
A small bowl;
A large bowl;
A comb/hair pick.

Directions: Fill the small bowl with about a handful of coconut oil. Meanwhile, fill the large bowl with some hot water, and then place inside the small bowl containing the coconut oil. Make sure that the small bowl is submerged in the hot water, not floating in it. Wait for the coconut oil to melt before dipping your fingers into it. Work the heated oil on your hair strands, starting on the ends and then gradually working up all the way to your roots. After coating all your hair strands with the oil, use the comb/hair pick to gently work out your tangled tresses. You may brush your hair and then style it as usual after making sure the coconut oil has thoroughly soaked in. Leave the oil on your hair instead of shampooing or rinsing it off – your hair will be nourished throughout the day this way.

3. Dandruff-free hair

Feeling defeated by your dandruff dilemma? It's time to defeat dandruff for a change with the help of coconut oil. Coconut oil has the ability to get rid of your itchy flakes as it also heals your scalp after taking a beating from different chemical-based conditioners, shampoos, colorants, and styling products. Say goodbye to dandruff for good with this recipe for making your own dandruff buster at home (this treatment is best done right before your bedtime):

Coconut Oil Dandruff Treatment

Materials: Two bowls (one should be larger than the other); a small towel; a large-toothed comb; and a jar of organic coconut oil (virgin).

Directions: Use a gentle formula shampoo to wash your hair strands, and then apply your conditioner as usual. Take the larger bowl and pour some hot water into it. Set the smaller bowl inside the larger bowl, and then fill the former with one scoop of coconut oil. See to it that the smaller cowl does not take on any of the hot water that is partially submerging it. Let the coconut oil liquefy as you start working the large-toothed comb on your hair strands to detangle them. Dip your fingers into the melted coconut oil, and then massage into your scalp using gentle strokes, making sure your entire scalp is coated. Once done, use the small towel to cover your oil-coated hair. Wash your hair the next day, following it up with an Epsom salt solution for best dandruff-busting results.

4. Protected hair color

You can use coconut oil as an excellent base in coloring your hair strands, since it can act as an effective medium in which to mix your hair coloring ingredients. The fact that coconut oil is able to work deep inside your hair strands easily in a shorter time assures you of getting the vibrant and long-lasting color you desire.

Coconut Oil Hair Coloring Base

Materials:

A jar of virgin coconut oil;
Two bowls (one should be larger than the other);
A separate bowl in which to combine your hair coloring ingredients;
Coloring herbs;
A shower cap;
A pair of gloves;
A large-toothed comb.

Directions: Start by pouring hot water into the larger bowl. Meanwhile, place about 2 to 3 spoonfuls of coconut oil into the smaller bowl before setting it inside the larger bowl (make sure the smaller bowl is partially submerged in the hot water). Wait for the coconut oil to melt before combining it with the coloring herbs. Apply the mixture to your hair strands and allow the color to set. Afterwards, wash your hair colored hair strands with a mild shampoo and lukewarm water (this helps remove any colorant as well as coconut oil residue). Use the shower cap to cover your hair overnight as you let the color continue to set.

5. Fast-growing hair

Letting your hair grow faster, thicker, and longer is possible with the use of coconut oil. Coconut oil naturally contains essential fatty acids as well as vitamins that leave your scalp healthy and nourished. Moreover, coconut oil helps eliminate any sebum that may have built up around your hair follicles.

Coconut Oil Daily Hair Nourishing Treatment

Materials:

Two bowls (one should be larger than the other);
A jar of organic coconut oil (virgin);
A large-toothed comb;
A small towel.

Directions: Use an all-natural formula shampoo to clean your hair before applying some conditioner and then detangling the strands using the large-toothed comb.. Meanwhile, fill the smaller bowl with two scoops of coconut oil before placing it inside the larger bowl that is filled halfway with hot water. Allow the hot water to melt the coconut oil before dipping your fingers into it. Work the coconut oil into your washed, detangled hair strands, making sure that the oil is massaged deep into your entire scalp. Leave the coconut oil on your strands overnight (use the small towel to cover your head before going to sleep).

6. Sun-protected hair

Protecting your vibrant hair from the damaging effects of the sun does not have to be difficult, especially if you have some coconut oil to help you do that. You can actually use coconut oil to make your own natural hair sunscreen, which you can use on your hair strands during those days when you will be more exposed to the sun.

Coconut Oil Hair Sunscreen

Materials:

A small bowl;
A large bowl;

Coconut oil, virgin, organic (1 jar);
A small towel or shower cap;
A hair pick or comb.

Directions: Take two to three scoops of coconut oil from the jar and place inside the small bowl. Meanwhile, fill the large bowl with some hot water (just enough to partially submerge the smaller bowl). Set the small bowl inside to allow the coconut oil to melt with the help of the hot water. Massage the coconut oil gently into your hair strands with your fingers. Afterwards, you can brush your sun-protected hair and then style it as usual.

CHAPTER 5

Having Better Health With Coconut Oil

How Coconut Oil Can Help You Achieve Amazing Health

Coconut oil isn't just for keeping yourself beautiful – it's also great when it comes to improving your overall health. In fact, populations that get most of their daily calorie intake from coconuts live a much healthier life than those that depend on other food sources. The Tokelauans which are part of New Zealand, for example, derive up to 62% of their calories from coconuts, and yet majority of their population have lowered blood pressure levels and low rates of coronary heart disease and diabetes.

If you are using virgin coconut oil, your body enjoys good cholesterol which contributes to healthy blood coagulation. It also gets a sufficient supply of antioxidants. Of course, your heart health gets a boost as well, with the reduction of blood triglycerides.

For this reason, you can gain a number of health benefits from coconut oil, benefits that go beyond improved immunity against diseases and infections, better digestion, and beautiful hair and skin. Coconut oil is able to you achieve the amazing health you desire with its different components:

Fatty acids (saturated). The saturated fatty acids that coconut oil contains, most of which are in the form of medium chain triglycerides, have the ability to be easily incorporated into the various systems in your body.

☐ *Lauric acid.* This type of saturated fatty acid makes up over forty percent of the entire saturated fatty acid content of coconut oil (capric acid closely follows). The body breaks down this fatty acid into a compound called monolaurin. Lauric acid and monolaurin helps prevent a wide range of infections, thanks to their ability to kill fungi, viruses, and bacteria.

☐ *Capric acid.* When capric acid undergoes a chemical reaction together with certain enzymes that are produced by some bacterial agent, it undergoes a transformation process that turns it into monocaprin, which has an effective antimicrobial property.

☐ *Caprylic acid + caproic acid + myristic acid.* These three types of saturated fatty acids found in coconut oil have high levels of antifungal as well as antimicrobial properties.

Polyphenols. Polyphenols are the components of coconut oil that are responsible for the latter's distinctive small and taste (virgin coconut oil contains high amounts of polyphenols).

Other components. The unsaturated fatty acids contained in coconut oil include linoleic acid and oleic acid; fatty acid derivatives include fatty esters, polyol esters, ethoxylates, polysorbates, monoglycerides, ethanolamide, and betaines; fatty alcohol derivatives include fatty alcohol ether sulphate, fatty alcohol sulphate, and fatty chlorides; and vitamins (E and K) as well as minerals like iron.

How to Use Coconut Oil to Achieve Amazing Health

Coconut oil has the power to function and benefit you as food as well as medicine in many different ways:

1. Whiter teeth and healthier gums

The reason why coconut oil is capable of improving one's overall dental health is that it helps improve the absorption of calcium in the body. This allows for the development of stronger teeth and the prevention of gingivitis and tooth decay.

If you want to have fresher breath and a healthier mouth, know that the Ayurvedic method of oil pulling can greatly reduce the amount of oral bacteria, which in turn reduces both plaque and cavities. To do oil pulling, simply put about a tablespoon of coconut oil in your mouth. Swish the oil around for about 15 to 20 minutes. After you expel the oil, you may brush your teeth. Keep in mind that it will be best to do oil pulling on an empty stomach – so doing it first thing in the morning may be a good idea.

Whiter teeth are a mere brush away – simply use a re-mineralizing toothpaste made with coconut oil to clean your teeth. Instead of relying on traditional toothpastes that may be made using some ingredients that are harmful to your oral health, consider making your own toothpaste with the help of this recipe for a coconut oil-based re-mineralizing toothpaste.

Coconut Oil-Based Re-mineralizing Toothpaste

Ingredients:

Coconut oil (3 to 5 tablespoons);
Calcium powder (5 tablespoons);
Baking soda (2 tablespoons);
Xylitol powder (3 tablespoons);
Mint essential oil (2 to 3 drops).

Directions: In a small mixing bowl, combine the calcium powder (you can process calcium tablets in a blender), baking soda, and xylitol by stirring well. Gradually add the coconut oil by drops into the mixture, followed by the mint essential oil. Once all the ingredients are incorporated, transfer the entire mixture into a clean glass jar. Simply dip your clean toothbrush into the re-mineralizing toothpaste, or dip a spoon or popsicle stick instead and then place the scooped toothpaste onto your toothbrush.

2. Acne-free face

Living acne-free can seem like a remote possibility for some; fortunately, coconut oil can be used to keep your face from breaking out. Coconut oil acts as an anti-inflammatory agent to minimize any redness, irritation, and other symptoms of inflammation brought on by acne.

It is important to keep in mind that coconut oil is not for everyone – it will still be best to do a patch test to check for allergies. However, if you have oily skin, you are likely to benefit greatly from using coconut oil. If you have used strong astringents in the past, you may have over-stripped your skin with its natural oils and that has prompted your pores to produce more oil, which can make acne worse.

Coconut oil can be very effective when it comes to drawing out most impurities that are lodged in your pores – the oil's ability to bind with the excess sebum along with the lipid-soluble dirt found on the surface of your skin, will help you remove all impurities from your pores. Keep in mind that those impurities are among the key reasons why you end up having acne and blackheads.

Using a gentle cleanser, wash your face first as you normally would. Afterwards, use your fingers to lightly apply coconut oil on your cleansed face in a thin layer (doing so also has an added moisturizing benefit to your skin). Make sure that the coconut oil has deeply penetrated into your facial pores before turning in for the night; otherwise, your bedding can get messy.

3. Soft and deodorized feet

Whether at work or during exercise, running around on your feet all day can leave them not only tired, but also rough, cracked, and smelly. Combat your feet woes by using coconut oil as a simple foot deodorizing and softening treatment. Right before bedtime, wash your feet thoroughly before using salt scrubs to exfoliate them gently. Rub a thick layer of coconut oil over your feet, and then cover them with thick socks. You will wake up the next day having softened, smoother, and pleasant-smelling feet. If you are suffering from athlete's foot, consider adding a few drops of tea tree oil to the coconut oil.

4. Healthier house pets

Coconut oil helps you have healthier house pets in more ways than one. You love your cats, but you hate their hairballs? Coating your house pets' paws with a small amount of coconut oil will help keep them from hacking up any hairball. You can also use coconut oil to keep your cats' as well as dogs' furs well-conditioned. Simply rub the oil through their coats to keep them healthier and shinier. This will also help relieve any itchiness to keep your pet from scratching the itchy area too much and irritating it (you will need to ask your pet doctor first before trying this). Finally, coconut oil can be used as a natural supplement to enhance or improve your pet's diet. After getting your pet doctor's approval, you can incorporate small amounts of coconut oil in your pet dog's or cat's food to help get rid of bad breath, maintain its ideal weight, and prevent any ligament and arthritis issues.

5. Protected against colds and flu

Protect your family members' health by encouraging them to take coconut oil daily. Coconut oil can help improve your immune system (it can increase your body's infection-fighting ability by helping increase the number of your white blood cells), which helps you and your family fight off colds and flu better. Thanks to the oil's antibacterial properties, it will be easy to ensure that your family stays protected from the spread of viral infection.

6. Chafing-free

Chafing usually happens when you rub fabric against your skin, which leads to soreness. Chafing may cause the skin to break or bruise, depending on the intensity of the rubbing. For those with sensitive skin, their inner thighs and groin areas might be prone to chafing as they walk. If you can use a lubricant on your skin to minimize the friction, then you can eliminate chafing altogether.

Coconut oil can be used to prevent chafing from taking place; simply rub it on the area prone to constant rubbing. When mixed with calendula, coconut oil can also be used as a soothing treatment for skin that has already suffered from too much chafing. And babies can have chafing-free skin as well with the help of coconut oil, especially in their diaper area. If your baby's bottom is already showing signs of irritation due to diaper rash, mix coconut oil into your diaper cream. To make your coconut oil chafing treatment, you can use the following recipe:

Coconut Oil Chafing Treatment

Ingredients:

Baking soda (1/8 cup);
Essential oils (4 drops of tea tree oil or lavender oil may work);
Arrowroot powder (1/4 cup);
Coconut oil (1/4 cup).

Put all these ingredients in a mason jar and stir well until they're thoroughly combined. Simply apply the mixture onto the affected area to relieve soreness and irritation.

7. Healed sore throat

Scratchy, sore throats can quickly be a thing of the past with the aid of some coconut oil thanks to its antibacterial and anti-inflammatory properties. In other words, it can attack the bacteria that's causing the sore throat – all while reducing irritation by working on the inflammation. Instead of reaching for a cough drop or syrup the next you suffer from a sore throat, try adding a small amount of coconut oil into your cup of tea, or simply taking coconut oil by the spoon. Alternatively, you can use the following recipe:

Coconut Oil Sore-Throat Concoction

Ingredients:

Coconut oil (2 tablespoons);
Lemon juice (3 tablespoons, freshly squeezed);
Raw honey (1/4 cup).

Combine these ingredients in a saucepan and heat them up on low heat. The goal is to melt the ingredients in order to combine them well together, not to cook them. Once the mixture achieves an even consistency, take a spoonful and ingest it as it is – or you can mix it with water if the flavor's too strong.

8. Relaxed and stress-free

Coconut oil is an excellent carrier oil for aromatherapy and massages since it can penetrate deep into the pores and get absorbed by the skin. Mixing essential oils and herbal extracts with coconut oil helps in making you feel the relaxing effect that you expect from massage or aromatherapy. At the same time, coconut oil also prolongs the shelf life of most organic massage and aromatherapy oils on the market. If you are using relaxation oils with coconut oil as base, you will also gain protection from bacteria, fungi, and viruses.

There is a good reason why it feels so relaxing to be lounging in a tropical beach that is surrounded by many coconut trees. The distinctive smell of coconut oil has a relaxing effect, which is why it is often used in aromatherapy. Simply massaging coconut oil onto your temples and into your scalp is enough to let you forget your stresses away – your headache will be gone and you will sleep better.

9. Lice-free

Eliminate pesky lice with the use of coconut oil, which is considered by a number of people to be effective in naturally keeping one's head lice-free. Coconut oil's saturated fat content is not only great for promoting healthy cholesterol levels and boosting energy, but also for removing lice. The reason is that the fat found in coconut oil suffocates lice. Aside from that, the fat makes it difficult for these parasites to hold onto hair. As long as you treated your hair with coconut oil, your hair strands will remain rather slippery to these minute bloodsuckers. The oil will also serve as an antibacterial solution, which you'll need to remedy possible skin infections and other dermal problems that may have been caused by lice.

Wash your hair first and then rinse with some apple cider vinegar. Allow your hair to air-dry before massaging the coconut oil into your hair strands and scalp. Cover your hair with a shower cap and leave the coconut oil on overnight. Simply run a comb through your hair in the morning before rinsing it out with water. Alternatively, you may use this guide in order to remove lice:

1. Heat up your stock of coconut oil to a comfortable temperature.

2. Coat your scalp with coconut oil.

3. Using a fine-toothed disposable comb, remove any nits that you may find in the hair's shaft.

4. Shampoo your hair with an organic shampoo bar.

5. Dry your hair completely with a towel (remember to wash your tower well after you use it).

6. Generously apply the heated coconut oil onto your scalp

7. Leave the oil in your hair for 12 hours. If you find it necessary, you can also have your head wrapped for 12 hours.

8. Use the fine-toothed comb in order to take away the dead lice.

9. Repeat this process as necessary – all lice should be removed with just two repetitions, but you can do more just to be sure.

10. Healed cold sores

Cold sores typically rely on the viruses that have caused them, and the only way to get rid of them as quickly as possible is to kill the causative agent. These sores are typically caused by a dormant strain of herpes virus, which are activated by illness, too much sun exposure, and anxiety or stress. These sores can be very uncomfortable, painful, or unsightly, and they can also be very slow to heal. Coconut oil can hasten the healing process by killing and inactivating the virus that caused them in the first place.

Coconut oil naturally has antiviral properties that allow it to effectively treat your cold sores and even treat fever blisters. Simply rub a tiny amount of coconut oil on the sore spot as well as the area around your lips. You can also take in 1 to 3 tablespoons of coconut oil daily to boost your immune system and get rid of the virus faster.

11. Protected from wound infections

Shallow wounds, cuts, scratches, and scrapes can be easily kept from being infected when you apply a sheer layer of some coconut oil over them. Coconut oil effectively works as a barrier against dust, dirt, and harmful bacteria.

Follow these tips to use coconut oil in preventing wound infections:

1. Get a sterilized dropper and fill it with coconut oil. Put a few drops into your ear canal if you have ear infection. Don't forget to lie still for a few minutes in order to let the oil into the ear canal.

2. Apply a coconut-based moisturizer to your skin after you shower. This will allow your skin to reestablish its pH balance and speed up healing.

3. If you have fungus infection, apply coconut oil directly to your fingernail for treatment.

12. Treated bug bites

Treat your bug bites as well as relieve any itchiness by covering the affected area with a few drops of coconut oil.

13. Calmed bruises

Coconut oil has been identified by a number of people to be effective in calming the area around bruises.

14. Cured yeast infections

Coconut oil has been found to be able to cure yeast infections when used topically or when taken directly, although you may have to ask your doctor first before trying it. Coconut oil contains caprylic acid, which is capable of breaking down the cell membrane of fungi. This prevents such microbes from multiplying and causing infection.

You can fight fungal infection internally and externally with coconut oil through the following methods:

1. Incorporate coconut oil in your diet – you may take in 3-5 tablespoons of coconut oil daily. You can start with a smaller dose and then gradually increase your intake.

2. Apply coconut oil on the infected area. Repeat twice or thrice a day until the infection is gone.

3. Create a coconut oil douche. You can do this by mixing coconut oil and distilled water. You can also use a coconut-oil-dipped tampon instead.

4. Use coconut oil with cinnamon oil. Apply a mix that contains equal parts of both oils on the affected area until the infection is gone.

5. Apply coconut oil with a few drops of vitamin E and garlic oil on the affected area. You can repeat this regularly until you have gotten rid of the infection.

6. Put oil capsules (2-3 should be sufficient) on the affected area before going to sleep. You can wear a pad to absorb the oil and prevent leakage.

15. Improved cholesterol levels

The lauric acid content of coconut oil gives it the ability to improve your cholesterol levels, which also helps your heart remain healthy.

16. Healthy and happy gut

A healthy and happy gut can be achieved with the use of coconut oil (upon your doctor's advice), which has been found to effectively soothe the occasional or chronic stomach issues such as IBS (irritable bowel syndrome), and it can also support regular bowel movement. Likewise, it relieves inflammation and aids in healing other disorders of the gastrointestinal tract. It even assists in destroying harmful bacteria that promote indigestion. You can also treat your ulcers by taking one tablespoon of coconut oil every day or including it in your dishes.

17. Cleared up nose

Clear up your airways with the help of a bit of coconut oil. You can make up your own vapor rub at home by combining coconut oil with rosemary and tea tree oils. You may then apply the mixture under your nose as well as on your chest – you can breathe more easily in a short while.

18. Protection from insect bites

Coconut oil makes for a good alternative if you do not want to use chemical repellants. This oil can be the base of an all-natural insect repellant to which you can add other herbs for a longer lasting effect.

Protect yourself from insect bites by mixing coconut oil with tea tree, peppermint, rosemary, or catnip essential oils. Apply the mixture as you normally would a commercial insect repellant. This homemade repellant will not only keep insect bites at bay, but it will also soothe the itchiness of any existing insect bites.

19. Cleaner ears

You can use coconut oil to get your ears cleaned: Simply wet (do not soak) a cotton swab with a bit of coconut oil, and then use it to gently remove the earwax from your ears.

20. Treated ear infection

If you are suffering from an ear infection, you can treat your pain symptoms (again, upon your doctor's advice) with the help of coconut oil's antiviral and antimicrobial properties; put a few drops of coconut oil into your affected ear canal. You can also add garlic cloves to coconut oil in order to come up with a stronger antibacterial solution.

21. Protected from nosebleeds

If you are suffering from frequent nosebleeds and you are certain that this is not caused by injury, then it is possible that it is due to dehydrated nasal cavity. This might happen during cold and dry seasons which cause the mucus membrane to crack and become itchy.

Letting your nostrils turn dry until they become irritated can lead to nosebleeds. Prevent your nostrils from being dried out by dabbing a little amount of coconut oil on the area inside your nose.

22. More comfortable breastfeeding

If you are breastfeeding your baby, make sure that you always carry with you a jar of coconut oil. Apply a small amount on your nipples to prevent them from becoming cracked and painful from breastfeeding.

In addition, incorporating coconut oil to your diet while breastfeeding will allow you to introduce the oil's nutritional benefits to your baby's diet. The fatty acids in coconut oil can also help you produce milk that can boost your baby's immunity against viruses and bacteria.

23. Improved metabolism

Give your metabolism a boost with the power of coconut oil. Add it to your dishes – the medium chain fatty acids of coconut oil are easily digested by your body, making it easy to convert by your liver into energy, which encourages your body to burn fat.

24. Sanitized dental accessories

Retainers, mouth guards, and other dental accessories are easier to clean and keep sanitized with the aid of coconut oil. It will help keep the bacteria and viruses from thriving in your accessories, thus preventing infection when you use such devices.

CHAPTER 6

Overcoming Stress with Coconut Oil

As you have learned in the previous chapter, it is possible to fight stress using coconut oil. If you're stressed all the time though, it's only expected that you are eager to get specific recommendations in creating your own concoctions. Well, in this chapter, you will discover essential oils that can be combined with coconut oil to create some of the most potent stress-busters.

1. Ylang Ylang

This flower is so effective in fighting stress that it actually boosts both cheerfulness and optimism. Some medical experts are even beginning to recommend Ylang Ylang to those who have problems keeping their blood pressure in check. Individuals with concerns regarding their serum cortisol levels can benefit from this aromatic oil as well.

2. Lavender

A common ingredient in bath and beauty products, this has a proven record in providing peace – eliminating problems such as irritability and anxiety. Its sheer potency has resulted to its use in some of the most unexpected scenarios, including calming patients in dental clinics and keeping those undergoing surgery sufficiently calm.

3. Rose

Much like the other entries in this list, rose has a scent that instantly calms the mind. Interestingly, however, this particular flower is believed to be most effective in fighting pregnancy-induced anxiety. It's for that very reason that pregnant women are sometimes told to soak their feet in warm water with a few drops of rose essential oil.

4. Frankincense

Popular among individuals who regularly meditate, frankincense is another potent anti-anxiety option. Despite often being associated with the spiritual, the scientific community is equally intrigued by this plant (specifically its gum resin). It was discovered in Keimyung University in Korea that frankincense has the power to reduce pain and depression, even among the terminally ill.

Combining Oils for Relaxation

So, how do you combine those essential oils with nature's elixir? It's quite simple. First, you will have to collect several things:

Dark, tinted glass bottles (approximately 10 milliliters in capacity);

Coconut oil (unrefined, pure, and organic);

Your preferred essential oil (choose one or many);

Plastic droppers (for transferring the oils).

Just put a few drops of your chosen essential oil into the glass bottle. Do note that the more you put in, the greater the calming effect of the resulting blend. Also, don't forget about the unique qualities of each oil. You should take your sensitivity into account as well. The usual minimum for these concoctions is 2 drops, with 40 drops being the maximum. Once you're done with that step, you pour coconut oil into the bottle. Be sure to leave enough space on top that the mixture won't spill over when you're getting a small amount with a plastic dropper. Feel free to try other essential oils. Likewise, don't hesitate to mix things up from time to time, especially when it comes to ratios.

Making Use of Stress-Relief Potions

The combinations you have created can be used in many different ways. For one, you could add a few drops to your bathwater before soaking in (make sure that it's warm though, since coconut oil has the tendency to solidify). Here's another option – put a small amount in a roller bottle and bring it with you. Whenever you feel stressed, simply pull it out of your bag or pocket and rub it on your palms (a little would be enough). Sniff the oil from your palm and you will soon enjoy complete tranquility. You could also put a small amount on your handkerchief if you wish to be more discreet.

Don't forget that the essential oils mentioned here aren't your only options. Try other oils firsthand and discover their synergistic effects with coconut oil. Don't be afraid to come up with your own unique blends, especially if you have very specific needs in your battle against stress.

CHAPTER 7

Fighting Diseases with Coconut Oil

Aside from providing those health benefits, coconut oil can also fight and prevent serious diseases. It's safe to say that no other household item can do the same. In this chapter, you will read about the scientific community's views and findings regarding nature's abundant elixir.

Reversing Alzheimer's Disease

Coconut oil is one of the best sources of medium-chain triglycerides (MCT), which allows for the production of ketone bodies through the body's metabolic processes. Together, MCTs and ketone bodies are a critical weapon against Alzheimer's disease – particularly by preventing the brain from starving.

How does this happen? A person's body uses insulin in order to convert the sugar that it derives from food, which is in turn converted into energy that the body can use. However, not all people have this very important ability – with diabetics being a good example. Because there is no insulin, the body is unable to produce the energy it needs. Eventually, the body will shut down because it does not have the necessary fuel to sustain itself.

A person's brain is capable of producing its own insulin, which this organ uses to produce glucose and fuel its own energy needs. However, since the brain creates its own energy like how the rest of the body produces glucose to sustain itself, the localized energy production also suffers the same risk as that of diabetes. That means that it is possible for the brain to stop creating its own insulin, and none of the glucose that passes through the brain is converted into fuel that will enable the brain to function. Without the necessary nourishment, the brain can literally starve to death.

Brain atrophy is one of the major problems that Alzheimer's patients suffer from, and it is practically the same atrophy that a diabetic's body goes through due to the lack of insulin. While a direct link between these two diseases is yet to be discovered, it's widely known that diabetics have a 65% higher chance of developing Alzheimer's compared to healthy individuals. For this reason, it is important for both diabetes- and Alzheimer's-afflicted patients to discover a way to fuel the brain and the rest of the body to prevent starvation or atrophy.

Fortunately, coconut oil can produce something that could serve as an alternative to glucose – ketone bodies. Not only do these ketone bodies create energy for the brain, they also promote blood flow to the brain. Likewise, they have a protective effect on neurons, making them even more valuable in preventing brain degeneration.

Preventing Diabetes

It is important to take note that cultures and countries that consume coconuts have lower occurrence of diabetes, compared to those that generally rely on polyunsaturated fats such as safflower oils and commercial vegetable oil. Coconut oil is able to make these people deal away with the need to eat too much carbohydrates in order to get the right amount of fuel.

Those suffering from diabetes can benefit from the ability of coconut oil to satiate hunger and cravings, as well as increase metabolic rates. For this reason, coconut oil is lauded for being able to curb type 2 diabetes, which is related to one's lifestyle and diet. The oil is also known to control type 1 diabetes, which is an autoimmune disease that locks down the ability to produce insulin.

Combatting Cardiovascular Disease

Among the major issues that revolve around the supposed dangers of ingesting coconut oil is that it may have ill effects on one's circulatory system. Because of thee oil's relatively high amount of saturated fat, some believe that it promotes heart disease and raises bad cholesterol levels.

Well, laboratory studies have proven that hydrogenated or refined coconut oil is the one that increases bad cholesterol, not natural virgin coconut oil. Also, coconut oil, regardless of type, does increase the total cholesterol in some individuals, but the rise is partly due to elevated HDL cholesterol (which is also known as good cholesterol). HDL is believed to be the kind of cholesterol that can protect you from heart disease.

Harvard Medical School studies revealed that getting 50% of one's dietary fat requirements (37% of total calories) from coconut oil does not lead to changes in total cholesterol (thus not increasing LDL or bad cholesterol) in healthy men. More importantly, coconut oil is the only fat in their study that is capable of increasing HDL in the body. Researchers from this institution even went as far as suggesting that regular consumption of coconut oil may improve blood lipid profiles and may eliminate the risk of developing cardiovascular diseases due to low HDL.

Demystifying the Antimicrobial Effects

John J. Kabara, along with other researchers, reported that particular fatty acids such as medium-chain fatty acids (MCFA) and other derivatives, have the capacity to combat viral, fungal, protozoal, and bacterial infections. When coconut oil is ingested into the body, the MCT is broken down into MCFAs and monoglycerides. This is also one of the reasons why MCTs found in human breast milk and some feeding formulas are very important in protecting the most vulnerable individuals against infection.

Antibiotics that can be purchased over the counter are only capable of protecting you from certain microbes, while the MCFA and monoglycerides that are abundant in coconut oil can kill a wide array of disease-causing agents that you may encounter on a daily basis. In fact, research shows that MCFA and monoglycerides can be very effective in killing off Chalamydia trachomatis, hepatitis C virus, streptococcus, and human immunodeficiency virus (HIV).

Simply put, coconut oil is an excellent household commodity as it makes sure that everyone in the family has the right tool in warding off infections.

Fighting Childhood Pneumonia

Antibiotic therapy, when virgin coconut oil is added to the treatment regimen, has been proven to become more effective in relieving symptoms of pneumonia. Children who were able to receive coconut oil therapy along with the prescribed antibiotics exhibit less wheezing, better oxygen saturation, and tend to stay in the hospital for a shorter amount of time.

Community-acquired pneumonia typically affect 34 to 40 out of 1,000 children in North America and in European countries, as reported by the American Academy of Family Physicians (AAFP). In the same vein, lower respiratory infections greatly contribute to childhood mortality in several developing countries. To date, community-acquired pneumonia is treated using intravenous administration of antibiotic ampicillin. In a study, some patients were given 2 milliliters of virgin coconut oil three days in a row. Respiratory rates normalized faster for patients with coconut oil added to their treatment. It was concluded that coconut oil may have amplified ampicillin's effectiveness because of the antimicrobial properties found in lauric acid, which coconut oil contains.

Curing UTI and Kidney Infection

Coconut oil has been traditionally and medically used to heal the body from urinary tract infection (UTI) and several other kidney infections. The MCFAs found in the oil serves as an all-natural antibiotic that destroys the lipid coating of bacteria, killing them in the process. At the same time, coconut oil also protects the liver from damage.

Here's an added benefit if you have a habit of storing coconuts in your household – if you drink coconut water, you will be able to hasten the healing process for damaged kidneys. Doctors even use coconut water as an injection to clear up kidney stones.

Preventing Arthritis and Reducing Inflammation

The high amount of antioxidants present in virgin coconut oil is proven to heal arthritis more effectively and reduce inflammation faster than most commercial medicines. In relation to that, coconut oil extracted using medium heat is found to have the ability to stop the formation of inflammatory cells, which makes this wonder oil as an effective anti-inflammatory and analgesic product.

Keeping Cancer at Bay and Assisting in Cancer Treatment

Coconut oil has two properties that make it effective as an assistive product in combatting cancer. First, the ketones produced upon digesting coconut oil do not feed tumor cells since they are dependent on glucose. For this reason, getting the necessary energy from coconut oil instead of other sources (this is typically done through a ketogenic diet), may help cancer patients recover faster.

Second, the MCFAs that coconut oil contains are capable of destroying bacterial lipid walls. This means that coconut oil greatly assists in the destruction of Helicobacter pylori bacteria which is responsible for amplifying the risk of getting stomach cancer. Even when cancer is chemically-induced, a dose of coconut oil can greatly help in preventing it from spreading.

Reducing Risks of Ulcerative Colitis and Stomach Cancers

One of the most common bacteria that can infect humans is Helicobacter pylori, which can be passed down from one generation to another. This bacteria is known for inhabiting the esophagus and the stomach, and is capable of producing excessive amounts of hydrochloric acid. This acid backs up into the esophagus, causing heartburn – or to use a more technical term, Gastro-Esophogeal Reflux Disease, or GERD. This reflux can cause gastritis, certain ulcers, and gastric cancer. On top of these, refluxes are also extremely painful. How does coconut oil do all these? Its lauric acid content can kill gut bacteria and fungi upon contact by destroying the cell wall.

CHAPTER 8

Healthier Baby with Coconut Oil

Coconut oil isn't just for health-conscious adults like you. It's also perfect for your baby – and no, this is not about the benefits that can be passed on through breast milk (as we have discussed in earlier chapters).

Cleaning Up Made Efficient

If you're having a hard time keeping your newborn clean, maybe you should try adding coconut oil to the equation. Unlike water, the oil is much more capable of dissolving and trapping dirt, meaning you won't have to wipe so much just to ensure that he's perfectly clean. Even meconium (an infant's earliest stool) is no match against coconut oil. Just put a small amount on a cotton swab and you are good to go. If you are feeling stingy, know that the oil (even in its purest form) isn't that expensive – especially if you compare it to other baby-friendly cleaning products on the market. Besides, it's guaranteed to be gentler than most of its commercially-made counterparts.

Defeating Diaper Rash, Naturally

If you have been caring for a baby, you know firsthand the trouble that diaper rash brings. Well, things are about to change for the better since coconut oil is a proven solution to that particular dilemma. Simply substitute diaper cream with coconut oil and you'll soon be saying goodbye to sleepless nights. The oil is the better choice here since it doesn't contain anything that could eventually end up irritating your baby's skin. Zinc oxide, for example, which is the most common diaper cream ingredient, is known to trigger allergies. It is also quite harmful if accidentally swallowed, and you do know that babies have the tendency to explore with their hands and put things in their mouth.

Solving the Case of Baby Acne

Baby acne does exist and surely, you don't want your little bundle of joy to have small, red spots on his face. Since most commercial products for acne are for teens and adults, you might give up on your quest to get rid of this dermal trouble. Actually, solving your problem is as easy as applying a small amount of coconut oil on your baby's face. Do it regularly for a couple of days and soon, it will be gone completely. If ever it does return, solving it again should not be hard. And given that coconut oil is among the safest substances, there's no need to think too much about possible long-term side effects.

Special Bath for Soft and Supple Skin

Although many associate babies with soft, supple skin, problems involving dryness do occur. Since it is not recommended to use commercial moisturizers and other similar products on an infant, you have to make use of a rather simple alternative – putting a few drops of coconut oil in your baby's bath water. You will be surprised at how effective this is, and the sheer convenience of this solution is just a bonus.

An Important Reminder on Sensitivity

It is a well-known fact that unrefined, organic coconut oil is virtually hypoallergenic, given how rare it is to find someone (regardless of age) who exhibits sensitivity reactions towards it. However, it would still be ideal to stay on the safe side and test your baby for possible allergies. Do a skin patch test before trying any of the suggestions in this chapter. Aside from that, if you notice anything unusual after you have applied coconut oil on your baby's skin, don't hesitate to get in touch with a physician right away.

CHAPTER 9

Boosting Brain Health with Coconut Oil

At this point, you are already aware of a great number of benefits that you can get out of using coconut oil as part of your diet or by applying it in different parts of your body. However, one of the most amazing things about coconut oil is that the medium-chain triglycerides (MCT) it contains can be used in repairing neural pathways and can positively impact memory and cognitive functioning.

Coconut oil can benefit people of all ages – you can start protecting yourself from diseases related to cognitive function, such as Alzheimer's and dementia, while you are still young. However, it's true that those in their golden years get the most benefit out of coconut oil's ability to improve brain functioning. If coconut oil is added to their daily diet with the right supplementary medication, then they are likely to experience a reversal of even the most crippling conditions of the brain.

Coconut Oil Improves Cognitive Ability

In one study, 20 subjects were randomly made to ingest either coconut oil or placebo during different days. Those that have taken coconut oil scored better on the Alzheimer's rating scale, meaning they have better cognitive performance. Here's something even more interesting – they were able to remember paragraphs better shortly after ingesting coconut oil. Take note however, that this is not a long and extensive study.

In 2009, Dr. Mary Newport's husband was able to come back from almost total dementia (and was able to finish tasks, recognize people, and remember events) just by consuming coconut oil. Dr. Newport is among the physicians who have tried to develop an Alzheimer's drug in 2004. They have tested the new drug through a clinical trial. It's important to note though, that her husband's condition was too severe to the point that he did not even qualify as valid subject.

Dr. Newport also observed that making patients take in coconut oil will only require caregivers to administer it twice a day, with doses given eight hours apart. The pharmaceutical drug, however, will have to be administered every three hours in order for it to work. That means that if Dr. Newport managed to get her husband into the clinical trial, then she could have lost him completely to the disease.

The reason why Alzheimer's patients greatly benefit from coconut oil is that this superfood is capable of producing ketone bodies when ingested. As explained earlier in this book, ketones are capable of serving as an alternative source of energy for the brain when it's unable to get enough glucose. In the absence of carbohydrates that typically fuel the brain, ketones become the reliable energy source that prevents the brain from starving.

Coconut Oil as a Cost-Effective Solution

At this point, people are looking forward to more developments about the use of coconut oil as a permanent solution when it comes to reversing the effects of dementia and Alzheimer's. While the research is not yet conclusive, it sure helps that coconut oil as a potential ingredient to a commercial drug has a non-patentable natural substance, which can be a driving point in lowering the cost of drugs that can be used to care for people with cognitive disorder.

Also according to the more recent studies, when the body is able to metabolize the MCT from the coconut oil, the ketones that it is able to produce may also be helpful in curing a variety of other diseases such as drug-resistant epilepsy, type 2 diabetes, brittle type 1 diabetes, multiple sclerosis, Parkinson's, and Huntington diseases.

It is also quite interesting to take note that Mr. Newport's dementia reversed itself over a year while he is taking in two doses of coconut oil in a day. He is able to run again, and experienced drastic improvement in reading comprehension and memory retention. His MRI results also showed that his brain atrophy has stopped completely.

CHAPTER 10

Choosing the Right Coconut Oil

What people know about fats and oils has drastically changed over the last decade. Unlike those in the past who have dismissed the possibility of using fats and oils in a healthy manner, today's populace is asking an important question – what kind of fat should people even be using? Those who've found the answer to that eventually ask another relevant question – since coconut oil contains the right kinds of fat, is it fine to use just any type of coconut oil?

Well, it is now time for you to get educated on how you can get the most out of nature's elixir by knowing how to buy one in the first place.

Dealing with the Brand Explosion

If you have been using coconut oil in the past, you may have noticed that the brands that carry coconut oil products have expanded exponentially. As a consumer, you may want to have a basic understanding of how these products differ from each other in terms of how they are farmed and processed. Right now, you also have to deal with middlemen and distributors, which can make the selection of which should go to your pantry even more difficult. Consumers will need to have a formula on what kind of oil is the best for them.

Here are some guidelines that you may want to follow in choosing the right oil:

1. Virgin vs. refined

There are two different types of coconut oil available on the market, namely virgin and refined. Refined oils are definitely less expensive but lack the coconut aroma and flavor. The reason for this is that they are extracted from copra, and thus they need to be bleached and deodorized. Unrefined coconut oil, also called virgin coconut oil, has a light coconut aroma and taste, which tend to differ from brand to brand. The taste and aroma will typically depend on the freshness of the coconut used and the type of processing.

If you want to get the most out of coconut oil, you need to look for the one that went through the least processing.

2. Processing method

Unrefined coconut oil has undergone cold pressing, a method in which oil is extracted from nuts and seeds at low temperatures (between 49 and 120 degree Fahrenheit). Most well-known companies are now paying attention to the freshness of the coconuts that they are using and are keen on having a quick turnaround time (from picking the coconuts, to bottling the product). They aim to keep the temperature as low as possible in order to preserve the nutritional integrity of the product. Also, do note that unrefined coconut oil is derived from fresh coconut meat.

Refined coconut oil, on the other hand, undergoes a rather complex process. In getting oil from copra (which is simply dried coconut meat), purification is the first step. This is done with the use of bleaching clays to get rid of most sediments that form due to drying. Afterwards, the resulting oil has to be exposed to high temperatures, as doing so is among the most reliable means of eliminating unwanted odor and flavor. The final step involves adding sodium hydroxide to ensure that the oil has a lengthy shelf life. Interestingly, some companies rely on chemical solvents to maximize the yield of copra. While it's definitely an economical move on their part, one has to question the downsides it brings – especially in terms of nutrition and long-term safety.

3. *Conventional versus organic*

Although coconuts don't often come into contact with pesticides and aren't being genetically modified by large-scale producers, it is still best to choose products that are produced organically. Not only are organically-grown coconuts healthier, they're also ecologically sound. In other words, they're grown through ways that ensure that the land will still yield healthy produce in the future.

4. *Glass or plastic packaging*

Here is something that you may want to keep in mind – food and plastic do not mix well when it comes to getting products that are designed to keep you in your optimal heath. While this is not a popular stance in this modern society, plastics are environmental disasters. At the same time, it is also important to keep in mind that food stored in plastic for a long amount of time may have toxicity issues, especially since you are dealing with a food product that goes through intense heat before it is bottled.

Of Considerations and Options

While most people will tell you that there is no need to nitpick on how a product is processed and packed, this notion does not really apply when it comes to choosing a health product like coconut oil. If you want to get the right coconut oil that you can use to improve your health, you will have to purchase virgin coconut oils that are grown organically and processed in the simplest way. You will also want them packaged in a glass jar.

Moreover, you should consider purchasing from companies known for providing fairtrade products. While this won't necessarily have an effect on your health, you'll at least know that those who have grown the coconut used for oil production have been properly compensated for their efforts.

Here are some choices that you can purchase in groceries and organic shops. Take note that all of these brands are virgin and organic, and are processed using cold-pressed raw methods or traditional small-batch pressing, which means that nutritional quality is kept intact:

1. *Maison Orphee Virgin Coconut Oil* – coconut came from the Philippines, and the company is from Quebec

2. *Alpha DME Virgin Coconut Oil* – coconut is from Solomon Islands, and the company is from British Columbia

3. *Nutiva Virgin Coconut Oil* – coconut is from Southeast Asia, and the company is from California

4. *Artisana Virgin Coconut Oil* – coconut is from Southeast Asia, and the company is from California

5. *Tropical Traditions Virgin Coconut Oil* – coconut is from the Philippines, and the company is from Wisconsin

Now that you know how to get the right coconut oil, you have the capacity to maximize its benefits. All you need to do now is to go over the tips mentioned in the earlier chapters of this book to start incorporating coconut oil in your life.

Conclusion

Thank you again for purchasing this book!

I hope this book was able to help you to become more enlightened about the many wonderful uses of coconut oil, which is why now is the right time to start viewing it as an essential food item, medicinal aid, and beauty tool to always have in your home.

The next step is to keep reminding yourself that even though there is no denying that coconut oil is of the best discoveries to apply to yourself and your family, it still pays to consider your doctor's advice and go signal first when using it for health purposes. You may be allergic to coconut oil, and regrettably suffer from its effects after applying it topically, ingesting it, or cooking with it.

You also have to take into account the fact that coconut oil is a type of fat, and that it does contain calories (about 9 per gram). When incorporating coconut oil in your daily diet, make sure to count the calories that it adds to your foods. You should also strongly consider using coconut oil as a substitute ingredient to your dishes, instead of happily adding it on top of every other fats or oils you use in cooking.

Finally, if you enjoyed this book, then I'd like to ask you for a favor, would you be kind enough to leave a review for this book on Amazon? It'd be greatly appreciated!

Thank you and good luck!

Anne